PROACTIVE COLOSTOMY DIETING GUIDE

Colostomy Cookbook On Easy Dietary Procedures On Slow Fiber Intake, Meal Plans And Recipes To Aid Body Digestion As You Experience Rapid Healing And Nourishment

DR. CHARLSE BLESSING

Copyright © 2023 by Dr. Charlse Blessing

~ 2 ~

DISCLAIMER

The information in this book is meant solely for educational reasons. This book's contents are not meant to be used in place of expert medical advice, diagnosis, or treatment. Any decisions you make about your health must be discussed with a licensed healthcare provider.

Every effort has been made by the author to guarantee that the material in this book is correct and current as of the date of publication. Still, since medical knowledge advances rapidly, new studies might be conducted that change our understanding this illness and how best to manage it with food.

This book may contains references to and mentions of various people, things, websites, organizations, and other entities that the author does not support, advocate, or have any association with. There is no implied sponsorship or collaboration; all references and remarks are made only for informational purposes.

In order to address their individual health concerns, readers are advised to independently verify any information contained in this book and to consult with healthcare specialists. Any negative effects arising from the use or implementation of the material in this book, whether direct or indirect, are not the responsibility of the author or the publisher.

The dietary suggestions and counsel provided in this book are broad in scope and might not be appropriate for every individual. Readers are recommended to seek tailored counsel from trained healthcare specialists as individual health problems and demands differ.

The reader accepts the conditions of this disclaimer by reading this book.

FACTS ABOUT THIS BOOK

The "Proactive Colostomy Dieting Guide" is a priceless tool that covers the intricate and varied path taken by those who have had colostomy surgery. This in-depth manual starts by giving a clear explanation of colostomy, revealing details about its several varieties, and assisting in a smooth transition to life with this medical modification. As the reader continues, the significance of post-colostomy nutrition is made clear, emphasizing the need to overcome nutritional obstacles, acknowledge the role that diet plays in healing, and develop a positive relationship with food.

One of the best things about this guide is its dedication to providing people with useful information. Choosing foods that are suggested, controlling portion sizes and meal scheduling, and maintaining nutrient balance are all covered in detail in the section on fundamental dietary guidelines. To help readers achieve optimal nutrition, the guide goes above and beyond by providing sample meal ideas, combining a variety of food categories, and helping them create well-balanced diet plans.

The need to be hydrated is emphasized for patients with colostomies, stressing the need to continue consuming fluids and offering advice on how to keep an eye on your hydration levels. Additionally, the guide tackles the complex issue of living with a colostomy by exploring weight control techniques, and activities specifically designed for individuals with colostomies, and avoiding typical errors that could impair general wellbeing.

Dietary limitations, allergies, and sensitivities are carefully taken into account, providing a personalized approach to the diet plan. Beyond focusing only on the physical side of recovery, the handbook also addresses people's mental and emotional health, offering coping mechanisms for difficult situations, creating support networks, and encouraging an optimistic outlook.

Sections of the guide that deal with real-world events, such as dining out and navigating social settings, provide more examples of how practical it is. It offers helpful advice on how to handle social events, eat out successfully, and explain dietary requirements. The handbook also includes important cooking and food preparation practices, with a focus on safe food handling, nutrient preservation strategies, and quick and simple recipes for a hassle-free cooking experience.

The guide's emphasis on holistic health is one of its best features; it covers topics like the value of vitamins and supplements, how to maintain regular bowel movements and travel advice for people who have colostomies. It discusses typical problems and offers answers, enticing readers to get expert advice when necessary.

Readers are encouraged to appreciate well-being and health as they work their way through this book. The last portion promotes adopting a proactive lifestyle, reflecting on accomplishments, and creating long-term health goals. The "Proactive Colostomy Dieting Guide" is essentially a lifeline, offering guidance and motivation to individuals negotiating the complex terrain of post-colostomy existence.

CHAPTER ONE

AN INTRODUCTION TO COLOSTOMY
Overview of Colostomy:

A colostomy is a surgical technique used to redirect the flow of stool from the colon to the exterior of the body by making an incision, or stoma, in the abdominal wall. This surgical procedure is usually carried out when diseases such as colorectal cancer, inflammatory bowel disease, or other disorders affecting the digestive system need the bypassing or removal of a piece of the colon. Waste can leave the body through the stoma and be collected in an abdomen-attached pouch once a colostomy is created.

A colostomy has a significant physical and psychological influence on a person's life. This operation can be performed on patients in an attempt to save their lives or to enhance their quality of life. People who are considering having a colostomy should know what the procedure entails, how it will affect their everyday lives, and how important it is to adjust to these changes proactively and constructively.

<u>Colostomy Types:</u>

Depending on the precise area of the colon involved and the position of the stoma, there are various types of colostomies. Ascending and descending colostomies are the two main varieties. feces from the ascending colon are usually diverted from the right side of the abdomen by an ascending colostomy, whereas the left side of the abdomen is used for a descending colostomy, which includes diverting feces from the descending colon. The underlying medical issue and the intended surgical outcome determine the particular type of colostomy that a patient will have.

Colostomies can also be permanent or temporary. Temporary colostomies are frequently made so that the colon can heal after an injury or sickness and then have the colostomy reversed. Permanent colostomies, on the other hand, are usually done in cases where reversal is not suggested or is not possible for medical reasons.

<u>Getting Used to Living with a Colostomy:</u>

Living with a colostomy requires adjusting to changes in one's physical, emotional, and way of life. People may first feel a variety of feelings, such as sadness, anxiety, and a sense of loss. Managing these feelings is an essential part of the process of adjusting. Being aware that a colostomy is an operation that can save or improve life will help one have a positive outlook during this period of transition.

Colostomy patients need to learn how to take care of their stoma and the skin around it. This includes learning how to change the pouch correctly, handle any issues that may arise, and

CHAPTER TWO

FOLLOWING COLOSTOMY SURGERY, NUTRITION IS CRUCIAL
Nutritional Difficulties:

A major medical treatment called colostomy surgery entails rerouting a portion of the colon to an opening in the abdominal wall, or stoma. Colostomy patients confront a variety of nutritional issues as a result of this life-altering procedure.

An immediate concern is the possibility of malabsorption of nutrients. Potential deficits could result from the altered intestinal anatomy's impact on the absorption of vital nutrients, such as vitamins and minerals.

Another important factor that is frequently influenced by colostomy surgery is fiber intake.

Although fiber is necessary for a healthy digestive system, some people may find it difficult to get enough of it because they are worried about possible blockages or irritation near their stoma. For those getting used to living with a colostomy, finding a balance between providing dietary demands and preventing problems is a tricky undertaking.

Another issue that people who have had colostomy surgery must deal with is staying hydrated. Dehydration is a common worry in this population, therefore people must be careful to ensure they consume enough fluids to prevent it. Changes in bowel habits and fluid absorption can affect hydration levels.

Furthermore, eating decisions may change as a result of coping with the psychological and emotional effects of having a colostomy. The total nutritional status may be impacted by restrictive eating patterns brought on by anxiety, aversion to particular foods, and body image issues. To tackle these obstacles, a thorough strategy that takes into account the nutritional needs following colostomy surgery from both a physiological and psychological perspective is needed.

Diet's Function in Healing:

A diet rich in nutrients and well-balanced is essential to the recuperation process following colostomy surgery. Sufficient nourishment is essential for immune system performance, wound healing, and general health. Particularly important for muscle preservation and tissue repair, protein is a staple of the post-colostomy diet. Lean meats, dairy, legumes, and other protein sources must all be consumed to encourage the best possible recovery.

Moreover, vitamin and mineral-rich diets are essential for promoting the body's healing processes. For example, zinc is essential for wound healing while vitamin C supports collagen synthesis and immune system function. A wider range of vital nutrients can be obtained by including a variety of fruits, vegetables, whole grains, and nuts, which will aid in a quicker and more seamless recovery.

Even though it's sometimes used cautiously, fiber is essential to a post-colostomy diet. Soluble fiber can be gradually added to assist control of bowel movements and avoid constipation without producing problems near the stoma. Maintaining digestive health and encouraging recovery requires finding a balance between fiber consumption and possible risks.

Furthermore, staying well-hydrated is crucial while the body is healing. Maintaining adequate hydration promotes healing, facilitates digestion, and helps avoid side effects like constipation. People ought to be motivated to keep an eye on how much liquids they consume and modify their intake according to their own needs.

<u>**Developing a Positive Connection with Food:**</u>

After colostomy surgery, establishing a positive relationship with food requires attending to the mental as well as the physical components of dietary decisions. Developing a positive attitude toward food and realizing the need for a well-balanced diet for general health and well-being are two important components.

In this process, education is crucial. Giving people knowledge about healthy food options, portion sizes, and the value of consuming a variety of nutrients gives them the power to make educated diet decisions. This information promotes a more inclusive and diverse diet and helps allay anxiety and fears associated with particular foods.

Recognizing potential emotional and psychological difficulties is equally crucial. Dietary decisions can be influenced by adjusting to changes in body image, social stigma fear, and concern about possible digestive problems. Facilitating transparent dialogue and providing assistance, including via therapy or support communities, can aid people in managing these affective facets and cultivating a constructive connection with food. Adding diversity to the diet is another way to encourage a positive relationship with food. Changing up the textures, flavors, and cooking techniques can add flavor and enjoyment to the post-colostomy diet. Positive thinking is aided by promoting the idea that food should be viewed as a source of enjoyment and nourishment rather than as a cause of limitation or fear.

In summary, establishing a positive relationship with food following colostomy surgery necessitates a comprehensive strategy that takes emotional, physical, and nutritional needs into account. In addition to recovering more quickly, people can have a happy and meaningful relationship with the food they eat by taking care of these factors.

CHAPTER THREE

FUNDAMENTAL DIETARY GUIDELINES FOR PATIENTS WITH COLOSTOMY
Harmonizing Elements:

For those who have a colostomy, maintaining a balanced nutritional intake is crucial because it greatly enhances general health and well-being. Keeping the right ratio of macronutrients, such as proteins, lipids, and carbohydrates, is one of the fundamental priorities. Patients with colostomies should prioritize eating a wide variety of foods to guarantee they get the vitamins and minerals they need.

The body uses carbohydrates as its main energy source, and choosing complex carbs like those found in whole grains, fruits, and vegetables can give you long-lasting energy without aggravating your digestive system.

Lean meats, fish, dairy products, and plant-based protein sources are important components of a diet since they are required for immune system function as well as tissue repair.

Nuts, avocados, and olive oil are good sources of healthy fats that are essential for maintaining organ function and enhancing the absorption of nutrients.

For those with colostomies, consuming enough fiber is also essential to maintaining a healthy nutritional balance. While soluble fiber sources are preferable to insoluble fiber, certain people may need to watch how much fiber they consume to avoid potential problems with intestinal obstruction or discomfort. Maintaining energy levels and promoting the body's capacity for healing and recovery are two benefits of maintaining the proper balance in nutritional intake.

Micronutrients including vitamins and minerals should also be properly taken into account in addition to macronutrients.

A healthy immune system and the ability to repair tissue are enhanced by vitamins A, C, and E, while calcium and vitamin D are especially crucial for bone health. A varied and well-balanced diet guarantees a complete and sufficient supply of these vital micronutrients, supporting the best possible health for colostomy patients.

Suggested Food Selections:

For colostomy patients, making the right food choices is essential to preventing problems and promoting overall digestive health. Rich in fiber, vitamins, and minerals, fresh fruits and vegetables are generally well-tolerated and promote general health. To find the fruits and vegetables that work best for their digestive systems, some people might need to try a variety of varieties.

Fish, poultry, tofu, and lentils are examples of lean proteins that provide vital amino acids without producing a lot of gas or discomforting the digestive system. Selecting cooking techniques like baking, grilling, or steaming that are gentle on the digestive system is advised. For calcium intake, dairy or dairy substitutes can also be added, while lactose intolerance may require selecting lactose-free products.

Whole grains are great sources of critical nutrients and long-lasting energy. Examples of these include oats, brown rice, and quinoa. These grains can help colostomy patients maintain a balanced diet because they are generally well-tolerated. Drinking enough water throughout the day is crucial to maintaining healthy hydration, which aids in digestion and guards against problems like constipation.

People who have a colostomy should consider potential trigger foods that could induce gas or discomfort in their digestive tract while making food choices. Maintaining a food journal can be a useful tool for seeing trends and choosing which items to include or cut out of your diet. All things considered, a diverse, nutrient-dense diet that is customized to each patient's tolerances is essential to their overall health.

Timing and Portion Management:

A proactive colostomy diet that incorporates portion control and meal timing is essential to the overall well-being and comfort of colostomy patients. By keeping the digestive system from being overburdened, optimal portion sizes lower the chance of pain, gas, or possible stoma problems. Patients with colostomies should prioritize eating smaller, more frequent meals throughout the day as opposed to larger, less frequent ones.

Maintaining a well-rounded diet without taxing the digestive system requires balancing the portion proportions of lipids, proteins, and carbs. In addition to improving digestion, smaller meals also lead to more consistent energy levels, which improves people's ability to maintain their general health. It's important to pay attention to your body's signals of hunger and fullness so that you can let it choose how much food is right for you.

Meal time is similarly crucial for patients with colostomies. Creating a regular eating pattern encourages regularity in digestion and aids in the regulation of bowel motions. Eating on a regular schedule helps the body become used to a predictable schedule, which is especially advantageous for people with changed digestive systems. Large meals should be avoided just before bed to minimize any potential pain during the night.

Additionally, observing the speed at which food is consumed can aid in improved digestion. Chewing food well facilitates digestion and eases the burden on the digestive tract. In addition to helping people better assess when they are full and attentive, slow eating also reduces the risk of overindulging and possible stomach problems.

To sum up, people with colostomies must practice portion management and thoughtful meal timing. This method helps people manage their colostomy through a proactive and long-lasting food plan that promotes digestive comfort, nutrient absorption, and general well-being.

CHAPTER FOUR

COLOSTOMY PATIENTS' MEAL PLANNING
How to Create a Diet Plan That Is Balanced

For people who have a colostomy, eating a balanced diet is essential since it promotes general health and helps manage any potential complications from the disease. Understanding the dietary requirements of colostomy patients and adjusting the intake of critical nutrients appropriately are the keys to creating a diet plan that works for them.

First and foremost, it's important to make sure you're getting enough fiber. Fiber helps to prevent constipation, which is a typical problem for those who have colostomies and encourages regular bowel movements. Including foods high in soluble fiber, like fruits, vegetables, and oats, can help the digestive system function more smoothly. Conversely, insoluble fiber, which is present in nuts and whole grains, can provide stool more volume and aid in the effective removal of waste.

Hydration is also essential for the proper management of colostomies. Dehydration can be avoided by maintaining adequate hydration, especially in light of possible fluid losses through the stoma. Melons, cucumbers, and soups are examples of foods high in water content that might increase fluid intake. It's important to keep an eye on each person's tolerance to different foods since some ostomy bag users may have flatulence or other problems after eating particular foods.

Lean protein consumption is crucial for tissue repair and general health in addition to these factors. Legumes, fish, poultry, and tofu are all great sources of protein that work well in a variety of dishes. Another thing to stress is portion control since smaller, more frequent meals could be more palatable than larger, less frequent ones.

In summary, careful consideration of fiber, water, and protein intake is necessary to provide a well-balanced diet for individuals with colostomies. Dietary modifications based on personal preferences and tolerances are essential for optimizing general health and reducing any difficulties related to colostomy.

Including Diverse Food Groups

To make sure that people with colostomies get a variety of nutrients that are vital to their health, it is crucial to diversify the food categories in their diet. Incorporating a variety of food categories into meals not only enhances their flavor and excitement but also improves their overall nutritional profile, promoting optimal health and averting nutritional deficiencies.

Rich in vitamins, minerals, and antioxidants, fruits and vegetables ought to make up a large portion of a person's diet. A spectrum of nutrients essential for wound healing and immune system function can be found in leafy greens, colorful vegetables, and a range of fruits. This is especially true for people who have had colostomies.

Another essential ingredient is whole grains, which offer fiber and complex carbs. Whole wheat products, quinoa, and brown rice can help control bowel motions and provide long-lasting energy. However, it's important to keep an eye on each person's tolerance to fiber because too much of it can cause pain in the digestive system.

Lean protein consumption is crucial for maintaining and repairing muscle. Diverse protein sources include fish, poultry, lean meats, and plant-based proteins like tofu and lentils. To make sure you get a wide range of important amino acids and other nutrients, it's a good idea to change up your protein options.

Dairy products, or dairy substitutes, are essential for maintaining bone health by supplying calcium and vitamin D. People who are intolerant to lactose may choose lactose-free substitutes or non-dairy sources high in calcium, such as fortified plant-based milk.

Lastly, adding necessary fatty acids that promote general health can be obtained by consuming healthy fats from foods like avocados, almonds, and olive oil. A complete nutritional profile is ensured by balancing the consumption of various food categories, which helps with colostomy management and enhances overall well-being.

Examples of Dinner Menus

For colostomy patients, creating enticing and nutritionally sound meal ideas is essential since it improves adherence to dietary guidelines and cultivates a positive relationship with food. A more pleasurable and sustainable eating experience is achieved by preparing meals that are not only delicious but also customized to meet dietary requirements and individual preferences.

A substantial, nutrient-dense, and high-fiber breakfast option is a bowl of oats garnished with nuts and fresh berries. A dollop of yogurt or a splash of plant-based or dairy milk improves the meal's flavor and nutritional content overall.

Lunch alternatives can consist of grilled chicken or tofu for protein, a vibrant salad with an assortment of veggies, and a side of full-grain bread or quinoa. A variety of vitamins and minerals are included when a wide variety of veggies are included, and the protein helps maintain muscle health and satiety.

Dinner may be steamed broccoli, sweet potatoes, and baked fish. Lean protein, complex carbs, and veggies are all balanced in this combo, making for a filling and well-rounded dinner. You can experiment with different herbs and spices to enhance flavor without sacrificing nutritional value.

A handful of mixed nuts, Greek yogurt with honey drizzled over it, or carrot sticks with hummus are a few examples of healthy snacks that can be included in a regular diet. These between-meal snacks offer a blend of fiber, protein, and good fats that help maintain energy levels.

It's crucial to adjust these meal ideas for sampling according to personal tastes, dietary constraints, and tolerances. Frequent consultation with a dietician or healthcare provider can assist in fine-tuning the food plan to suit the unique requirements of every colostomy patient.

CHAPTER FIVE

HYDRATION FOR PATIENTS WITH COLOSTOMY
The Value of Hydration

Maintaining the general health and well-being of individuals with colostomies is greatly dependent on enough hydration. Maintaining proper fluid balance is essential for many physiological processes in people with colostomies, in which part of the colon is diverted to the abdominal wall. After colostomy surgery, the digestive system may experience major changes. It is even more important to maintain enough hydration levels to support these adaptations.

Preventing dehydration is one of the main reasons to emphasize hydration—a condition that can result in several difficulties. Patients with colostomies who are dehydrated may experience thicker, more difficult-to-pass feces, which raises the possibility of stoma obstructions. Furthermore, if electrolyte imbalances caused by dehydration are not treated, the body may become less able to regulate vital minerals, which may result in weakness, exhaustion, and even more serious problems.

Sufficient hydration not only avoids difficulties but also improves the digestive system's effectiveness. Drinking plenty of water supports the body's attempts to absorb and use nutrients from food, including vitamins and minerals. For patients with colostomies, in particular, maintaining appropriate nutritional status is critical for overall health and post-surgery recovery.

Additionally, maintaining kidney function and reducing urinary tract infections are two benefits of staying hydrated. Maintaining enough fluid levels helps to flush out toxins and prevents the production of concentrated urine, which can lead to infections. Urinary tract issues may be more common in patients who have had colostomies.

Staying hydrated is beneficial for controlling the consistency of ostomy output when using a colostomy. Drinking enough water can help keep the stool consistency balanced, which makes managing the stoma easier and reduces the risk of leaking or skin irritation near the stoma site.

In conclusion, colostomy patients must stay hydrated. It is fundamental to the prevention of problems, the support of digestive function, and the enhancement of general health and well-being.

Fluid Consumption Suggestions:

When deciding on the right fluid intake, people with colostomies must carefully take their lifestyle, medical history, and unique characteristics into account. Although there are broad suggestions, it is essential to customize fluid intake recommendations to each patient's unique needs to maximize health outcomes and avoid issues related to dehydration.

Regarding colostomy, the daily recommended fluid intake generally corresponds with normal recommendations for the general population, which generally prescribe eight 8-ounce glasses of water per day. It's crucial to understand that each person's needs may differ according to their age, weight, degree of exercise, climate, and general health.

Patients who have colostomies should be encouraged to drink more than just water. Drinking hydrating drinks such as clear broths, diluted fruit juices, and herbal teas can help satisfy daily fluid requirements. It's important to remember that, although they increase fluid consumption overall, alcoholic and caffeinated beverages may have diuretic effects and should only be used in moderation.

Urine output monitoring is a useful way to determine one's level of hydration. Dehydration may be indicated by dark or concentrated urine, necessitating a higher fluid intake. Conversely, light-colored pee frequently denotes sufficient hydration. However it's important to remember that some drugs or illnesses can affect urine color, so constant contact with medical professionals is necessary for an accurate diagnosis.

Healthcare providers and colostomy patients can work together to provide customized recommendations for fluid consumption. Keeping a hydration notebook to record fluid intake and output might help identify trends and modify recommendations. Following up with medical professionals regularly can assist in keeping an eye on a patient's level of hydration and modifying the recommended daily intake of fluids as needed to accommodate changing needs.

To achieve appropriate hydration and general well-being, fluid intake recommendations for patients with colostomies should essentially be customized, flexible, and routinely reevaluated.

Tracking the Level of Hydration:

A vital component of proactive colostomy care is monitoring water levels, which enables patients to preserve their best health, avoid difficulties, and guarantee the efficient operation of their digestive system. Patients with colostomies, in particular, must pay close attention to their level of hydration to reduce the dangers of dehydration and its possible effects on stoma function and general health.

Observing the color and output of urine is a useful way to track one's level of hydration. Urine that is clear or light in color usually suggests enough hydration, but urine that is black or concentrated may indicate dehydration. Urine color can be affected by certain medications and medical problems, so it's vital to keep that in mind. For a more precise evaluation, any apparent alterations should be reviewed with healthcare professionals.

Keeping a daily log of your fluid consumption can be a useful tool for tracking your level of hydration. Monitoring the kinds and volumes of fluids ingested as well as any variations in stoma output gives a complete picture of a person's level of hydration. At routine check-ups, this information can be given to medical practitioners, enabling recommendations for fluid consumption to be modified in light of the patient's particular needs and circumstances.

Healthcare professionals may use clinical assessments in addition to self-monitoring to determine hydration levels. Tests on the blood that assess kidney function and electrolyte levels can reveal important information about the body's level of hydration. Frequent meetings with medical professionals guarantee that any new difficulties about dehydration can be handled quickly, avoiding complications and enhancing general health.

Additionally, individuals with colostomies must get education regarding the warning signs and symptoms of dehydration, which include increased thirst, dry mouth, dark urine, weariness, and dizziness. Early detection of these signs enables people to take preventative action against dehydration, such as drinking more fluids or getting help when needed.

In summary, keeping an eye on one's hydration levels is a complex and dynamic process that calls for both independent assessment and cooperation from medical experts. Colostomy patients can improve their quality of life and maximize their health outcomes by being proactive and cautious when it comes to controlling their hydration.

CHAPTER SIX

MANAGING WEIGHT AFTER COLOSTOMY SURGERY
Healthy Weight Goals after Colostomy Surgery:

Reaching and maintaining a healthy weight following colostomy surgery is essential for general well-being and a speedy recovery. One of the most important aspects of post-colostomy treatment is setting achievable and realistic weight goals. It's critical to understand that each person's weight objectives may differ depending on age, underlying medical issues, and the kind of surgery they had.

The necessity to promote the healing process while avoiding undue physical stress on the body is a major factor to take into account while establishing healthy weight goals.

Rapid weight gain or reduction may affect the stoma and its surroundings, thereby complicating matters.

A balanced diet that contains the necessary nutrients to support healing is crucial in this process, and nutrition plays a major role in it.

To set individualized weight targets, it's best to collaborate closely with medical professionals, such as nutritionists and surgeons. These objectives could entail a mix of dietary changes, consistent exercise, and continuous progress tracking. For people with colostomies, restoring their health and improving their quality of life requires finding a balance between maintaining a healthy weight and making sure they are getting enough nourishment.

Achieving a healthy weight involves more than just physical factors; psychological well-being is as important. A key element of the post-colostomy journey is cultivating a sense of self-acceptance and embracing a good body image. This all-encompassing strategy for managing weight promotes a more satisfying and long-lasting healing process.

Activities for Patients with Colostomy:

An essential part of post-colostomy care is doing the right exercises, which improves both physical and mental health. Although specific circumstances should inform exercise suggestions, there are broad guidelines that people with colostomies can take into consideration to support an active and healthy lifestyle.

Colostomy patients can gradually add low-impact exercises like walking, swimming, and stationary cycling to their program as they are often well-tolerated. These exercises strengthen the heart without putting undue strain on the stomach region. Exercise for strengthening the core muscles can aid with stability, and posture, and lower the risk of surgical site problems.

To encourage flexibility and relaxation, yoga and mild stretching activities are helpful. These exercises can be modified to meet each person's comfort level and post-operative recuperation. Seeking advice from medical experts, such as physical therapists, is crucial if you want customized workout plans that fit each colostomy patient's unique demands and restrictions.

After colostomy surgery, consistency is essential to continuing an active lifestyle. Long-term success is influenced by gradual advancement, consistent monitoring, and modifying training regimens as necessary.

A safe and successful fitness regimen for colostomy patients also includes maintaining hydration and being aware of the body's signals while exercising.

Preventing Typical Weight Loss Mistakes:

After colostomy surgery, managing weight demands a deliberate and knowledgeable technique to steer clear of typical errors that could impede recuperation and general well-being. The urge to follow rigid eating regimens or drastic diets to lose weight quickly is a common problem. Such activities have the potential to significantly affect the stoma and general health by compromising the nutritional intake necessary for healing and possibly resulting in deficits.

The possibility of dehydration is another danger to be aware of. For those who have a colostomy, maintaining adequate hydration is essential because it helps avoid problems like constipation and dehydration, which can impair weight control and general health. Patients with colostomies should make drinking water a priority and keep an eye on their fluid balance, particularly when exercising.

Emotional health and weight control are intimately related, and harmful habits can be exacerbated by stress or anxiety. Getting help from medical specialists, support networks, or mental health services can help with emotional difficulties and cultivate an optimistic outlook.

And last, it's imperative to refrain from contrasting one's weight control journey with that of others. Every person's road to recovery is different, and variables like age, health history, and surgical details matter a lot. After colostomy surgery, achieving modest victories, keeping a patient and optimistic mindset, and concentrating on personalized goals all help to make weight management more successful and long-lasting.

CHAPTER SEVEN

PARTICULAR THINGS TO TAKE INTO ACCOUNT WHEN FOLLOWING A DIET
Taking Care of Dietary Restrictions

Considering dietary restrictions is an essential part of creating a thorough and useful Proactive Colostomy Dieting Guide. others who have colostomies encounter particular difficulties, and they may require very different diets than others who do not have them. With the altered digestive system and possible allergies, it is necessary to design a diet plan that meets certain constraints while still providing critical nutrients.

It is essential to comprehend the patient's medical background and the reasons behind the colostomy to customize an appropriate diet. Restrictions on particular food groups or textures may be necessary for some conditions to avoid problems or pain. For example, if the inflammatory bowel condition caused the colostomy, then consuming high-fiber foods may need to be reduced to prevent irritation. On the other hand, if colorectal cancer causes colostomy, the emphasis might be on sustaining ideal nutrition to support general health while recovering.

Furthermore, taking into account possible drug interactions is crucial while managing dietary limitations. The diet plan needs to be modified by the possibility that some medications may affect how particular nutrients are metabolized or absorbed.

It is imperative to engage in collaboration with healthcare specialists, such as dietitians and gastroenterologists, to guarantee that dietary recommendations are in line with an individual's medical management and overall health.

Furthermore, education is essential when it comes to dietary restrictions. Giving colostomy patients comprehensive knowledge about how various meals affect their digestive tract gives them the power to make wise decisions. Advice on portion management, cooking techniques, and substitute ingredients that can be used in their diet without endangering their health may be included in this.

Allergies and Sensitivities:

Creating a Proactive Colostomy Dieting Guide becomes much more complicated when considering allergies and sensitivities. A colostomy's changed gut anatomy may make a person more prone to certain allergies or sensitivities. To avoid negative responses, it may be necessary to approach common allergens like dairy, gluten, and nuts cautiously.

A complete evaluation of the patient's medical history, including any prior allergies or intolerances, is necessary for the identification and management of allergies and sensitivities. Moreover, those who had a colostomy due to a particular medical condition, such as Crohn's disease, might be more sensitive to particular foods that worsen their symptoms.

According to the Proactive Colostomy Dieting Guide, careful consideration should be given to the selection of ingredients and food preparation. To guarantee a varied and well-balanced diet, this entails presenting comprehensive lists of possible allergies in different food categories along with replacements or alternatives. For instance, lactose-free or plant-based substitutes can be suggested to someone with a dairy allergy to satisfy their dietary requirements without causing negative side effects.

Furthermore, people with allergies or sensitivities must have constant contact with medical professionals. Frequent examinations can help track any changes in sensitivity over time and enable diet plan modifications as necessary. Working together with nutritionists and allergists guarantees a comprehensive strategy for managing dietary restrictions and allergies in the setting of a colostomy, supporting general health and digestive health.

Tailoring the Dietary Program:

A Proactive Colostomy Dieting Guide's foundation is customized diet planning, acknowledging that a one-size-fits-all strategy is insufficient for people with different medical backgrounds, dietary requirements, and lifestyle choices. Customization is essential to meeting the distinct needs and objectives of every colostomy patient, guaranteeing that dietary guidelines correspond with their situation.

To properly tailor the diet plan, a thorough evaluation is carried out, accounting for variables like age, gender, weight, degree of exercise, and underlying medical issues. For example, the nutritional needs of an older person with a colostomy may differ from those of a younger person. To maintain optimal health and energy levels, dietary modifications may be required.

Customization also entails adjusting the diet plan to correct for any excesses or shortfalls in the person's existing nutritional state. To determine specific nutrient demands, such as vitamin and mineral levels, and to guide modifications to the meal plan accordingly, blood tests and routine health checks are essential. This guarantees that the person gets the proper ratio of nutrients to aid in healing, avert problems, and improve general health.

Customization in the context of a colostomy also includes resolving certain digestive difficulties. The eating plan can be modified to successfully control any bowel habit changes or increased gas production that certain individuals may encounter. To maximize digestive comfort, this may entail suggesting foods that are readily digested, adding probiotics, or adjusting fiber consumption.

Additionally, a personalized diet plan takes into account cultural and personal preferences, understanding that following dietary guidelines is more likely when the plan fits the person's preferences and way of life. The long-term sustainability of the tailored food plan is ensured by close collaboration with healthcare specialists and the individual's involvement in the decision-making process.

CHAPTER EIGHT

EMOTIONAL AND MENTAL HEALTH
Coping Mechanisms for Emotional Difficulties:

Adopting a proactive approach to a colostomy diet requires major mental obstacles in addition to physical adjustments. After colostomy surgery, patients frequently experience anxiety, depression, and a change in how they view their bodies. Coping mechanisms are essential for getting over these emotional obstacles.

Promoting open communication is a crucial coping mechanism. Emotional burdens can be reduced by discussing feelings and concerns with a family member, trusted friend, or mental health professional. It's important to recognize and embrace the emotions that come to the surface.

Through this technique, people can examine their emotions without passing judgment, creating a more positive emotional environment.

Additionally, using relaxation and mindfulness practices can have a transforming effect. People can learn to manage their emotions again by practicing yoga, meditation, or deep breathing. They can focus on the here and now with mindfulness, which lessens their concern about the past or the future.

Furthermore, education is essential for emotional functioning. Being aware of the colostomy procedure, its aftereffects, and the possible advantages of a proactive diet plan enables people to take control of their health. A sense of control is fostered by knowledge, which lessens the fear of the unknown.

Participating in colostomy support groups offers a special forum for exchanging experiences. Making connections with people who have had comparable difficulties promotes a feeling of solidarity and normalizes emotional hardships. It can be very comforting to hear about peers' successes and coping mechanisms.

Finally, it's critical to strike a balance between social interactions and self-care. Setting aside time for enjoyable and soothing pursuits, such as hobbies or quality time with loved ones, is beneficial to mental health in general. Through the proactive application of these coping skills, those starting a colostomy diet can effectively manage emotional obstacles with fortitude and an optimistic outlook.

Resources and Support Systems:

Starting a proactive food plan for colostomy requires a strong support network and access to helpful information. Acknowledging the significance of these components is crucial for those undertaking this life-changing experience.

The participation of friends and family is the cornerstone of any successful support system. Their comprehension, encouragement, and emotional support can have a big impact on the person's mental health. In these partnerships, being able to share worries, fears, and victories through open communication helps to build a sense of connection.

Another source of help is joining colostomy support groups. These communities provide a forum for people to talk about their experiences, give and receive counsel, and get support from others who have been through similar circumstances. Online communities and forums give people in the digital era a place to connect with a wide variety of people worldwide and offer a virtual area for ongoing support.

Having access to medical experts is essential for negotiating the intricacies of colostomy diet plans. Working together with medical professionals guarantees tailored advice, taking care of particular dietary requirements, and keeping an eye on general health. Consultations with a healthcare team regularly provide a proactive way to handle any issues that might come up during the dieting process.

Apart from one's assistance, people gain from instructional materials. Thorough manuals, reliable websites, and literature on colostomy dieting provide people with the information they need to make educated food decisions. Nutritionists with expertise in colostomy care can offer customized guidance, enhancing the dietary experience.

Resources are made available through the substantial contributions of governmental and nonprofit organizations that specialize in colostomy treatment. These groups frequently provide community activities, financial aid programs, and educational materials. By utilizing these resources, one may establish a comprehensive support system that gives people the knowledge and resources they need to follow a proactive and successful colostomy diet plan.

Developing an Upbeat Attitude

A proactive colostomy dieting guide's transforming element is creating and sustaining a good mindset. After colostomy surgery, a person's mental attitude has a significant impact on their capacity to adjust to changes, overcome obstacles, and accept a new way of life.

Self-compassion is essential to cultivating a good outlook. Being aware that every trip is different and could have highs and lows enables people to treat themselves with kindness while going through the process. Resilience and optimism are enhanced by acknowledging and appreciating modest accomplishments as well as accepting faults.

Cultivating positivism also requires setting reasonable goals. Instead of concentrating on large-scale successes, people might divide their goals into doable milestones. This strategy makes it possible to feel successful at every turn, which strengthens positive thinking and inspires perseverance.

Gratitude and mindfulness exercises are essential for developing an optimistic outlook. A person's general well-being is influenced by their ability to be in the present moment and to see and value the positive aspects of life. Daily appreciation practices help cultivate an attitude of thankfulness for the body's resiliency and the capacity to initiate proactive colostomy diets.

A growth mentality is essential for overcoming obstacles. Resilience is fostered when setbacks are viewed as chances for growth and learning rather than as insurmountable barriers. This change in perspective enables people to view the colostomy diet plan as a dynamic process and respond to modifications positively and proactively. One of the most potent catalysts for a happy outlook is social support. Having supportive people around oneself, whether they be family, friends, or support groups, fosters an optimistic atmosphere. By encouraging one another via shared experiences and setbacks, a sense of community is formed and the idea that the colostomy diet guide is a trip that is taken together is strengthened.

To sum up, cultivating and maintaining a good outlook is a continuous effort that is integrated with the practical elements of a proactive colostomy diet plan. People can travel through this path with resilience, optimism, and a sense of empowerment by embracing a growth mindset, practicing mindfulness, implementing self-compassion, setting realistic goals, and cultivating social support.

CHAPTER NINE

DINING OUT AND MANAGING SOCIAL CIRCUMSTANCES
Getting Around at Social Events:

For those who have a colostomy, attending social events may be both fun and difficult. To ensure comfort and confidence, it is important to take preemptive measures. The secret to handling these circumstances well is good communication.

To begin with, educate your close friends and family about your food requirements and colostomy to build their understanding and support. If you plan to attend a larger gathering, think about contacting the host ahead of time to discuss possible accommodations and food alternatives. This lets you make plans in advance and guarantees that your dietary needs are met.

It's important to keep a positive attitude and not let your colostomy issues overshadow the occasion while you're in social settings. If someone asks you about your disease, take advantage of the chance to clear up any confusion and raise awareness. Additionally useful for breaking the ice and putting people at ease around you is a sense of humor.

Additionally, consider what you're wearing. Your comfort and confidence can be increased by dressing in a way that makes accessing your colostomy pouch simple. Select clothing that not only fulfills your necessities but also gives you a positive self-image.

Keep in mind that social circumstances might change, therefore flexibility is essential. Keep the essentials in a tiny bag so you can covertly handle any problems without attracting undue attention. People who have a colostomy can engage in a variety of events with confidence by being open, communicative, and proactive, which promotes a sense of inclusion and connection.

Tips for Eating Out:

For people who have a colostomy, dining out might provide special obstacles, but it is possible to enjoy restaurant meals without sacrificing comfort with proper planning and knowledge. First, do some prior research on eateries to find those who are willing to make alterations or have flexible menus. Don't be afraid to contact ahead and discuss your preferences; many businesses are willing to alter dishes to accommodate special dietary requirements.

When looking through the menu, concentrate on foods that are well-cooked and easily digested. Avoid meals that could irritate or create discomfort, and if you want to avoid overeating, think about consuming smaller portions. Safe options generally include soups, grilled proteins, and well-cooked vegetables.

Furthermore, exercise caution when consuming highly seasoned or spicy foods as they might not be suitable for your digestive system.

When dining out with a colostomy, timing is everything. Arrange your meals to align with your body's innate rhythm, steering clear of circumstances that can compel you to eat rapidly or in a hurry. Inform the server of any dietary requirements you may have, stressing the value of easy preparations and avoiding particular substances.

Keep a covert supply kit with the essential colostomy supplies on hand in case something unforeseen happens. Having this equipment on hand gives you peace of mind so you can enjoy your meal without worrying about unneeded things. People with colostomies can enjoy eating out while putting their digestive health first by choosing restaurants carefully, choosing menu items carefully, and efficiently interacting with staff members.

Effectively Communicating Dietary Needs:

A key component of proactive colostomy care is effectively conveying dietary demands, which guarantees that people can enjoy meals without sacrificing their well-being. Create a succinct and understandable description of your dietary needs first, emphasizing any particular foods or ingredients that can cause problems. To foster a friendly environment, distribute this information to your usual dining companions, family, and friends.

Don't be afraid to let restaurant employees know what you need when you're eating out. If they are informed of dietary requirements, servers, and cooks frequently satisfy them. Be firm yet courteous, stressing the value of easy recipes and steering clear of particular components.

Making suggestions or other options available can help the process go more smoothly for everyone.

If you travel a lot or eat in culturally varied situations, always have a dietary card with you that lists your requirements in several languages. You can discreetly give the server this card to ensure that they fully grasp your needs, even in cases when there may be a language issue.

Inform people close to you about your food requirements and colostomy in social settings. Promote candid communication and respond to any inquiries that may come up. Being open and honest about your illness promotes understanding and an inclusive environment where others are considerate of your special needs.

Remember that communication is two-way. Be open to hearing others' questions and concerns, and take advantage of the chance to debunk any misunderstandings or myths regarding the management of colostomies.

Through proactive and transparent communication, people with colostomies can establish a network of support that helps them to confidently and easily navigate social situations and dining experiences.

CHAPTER TEN

TECHNIQUES FOR COOKING AND PREPARING FOOD
Proper Food Handling for Patients with Colostomy:

People who have a colostomy must make sure they handle food safely because their digestive systems have changed significantly. Maintaining good hygiene and handling food correctly can help avert issues and enhance general health. Cleaning should come first; hands should be properly cleansed both before and after handling food. By doing this, the possibility of bringing dangerous germs into the digestive tract and perhaps causing illnesses is decreased. To keep the atmosphere hygienic, all utensils, cutting boards, and surfaces need to be cleaned regularly.

Patients with colostomies should watch what they eat to reduce the possibility of digestive problems.

Avoiding raw or undercooked meats, raw shellfish, and unpasteurized dairy products can help reduce the spread of bacteria. Fresh produce needs to be well-cleaned, and the expiration dates of pre-packaged goods need to be verified.

Another essential component of handling food safely is portion control. Patients with colostomies may be able to better control their digestion by eating smaller, more frequent meals. This lessens the burden on the digestive system in addition to assisting with the absorption of nutrients. Other precautions that help keep colostomy patients' diets safe and nutritious include minimizing cross-contamination, storing leftovers appropriately, and promptly refrigerating perishable goods.

Making sure that meals are prepared with the needs of the colostomy patient in mind is crucial when interacting with others in social situations and communicating dietary restrictions. People who have colostomies can minimize the risk of issues while still enjoying a varied and nutritious diet by adopting these safe food handling techniques into their daily lives.

Techniques for Cooking to Preserve Nutrients:

Cooking for people who have a colostomy requires not just making sure the food is safe, but also retaining vital nutrients that promote general health. The selection of cooking techniques is essential for maintaining the nutritional content of ingredients. The best techniques include steaming, roasting, and microwaving since they cook food more quickly and at a lower temperature than boiling or frying.

Because steam cooking preserves the original aromas and colors of fruits and vegetables, it is very excellent at keeping nutrients in food. For colostomy patients who want to get the most out of their meals in terms of nutrition, this strategy minimizes nutrient loss.

Another technique that might improve food's flavor and nutritional content is roasting. Roasting preserves vital vitamins and minerals by cooking food in their juices. To keep the food nutritious and easily digested, use small amounts of oil and stay away from overseasoning.

A quick and practical method that keeps nutrients well is microwaving. Reduced heat exposure and brief cooking durations help to retain nutrients. However, since dangerous chemicals could seep into the food, it's imperative to avoid using plastic containers that aren't marked as microwave-safe.

On the other hand, because many vitamins are water-soluble and might leak into the cooking liquid, boiling could result in nutrient loss. Deep-frying in particular should be done carefully since it can increase unneeded fat content and lower the nutritional value of the dish.

Colostomy patients can have a healthy, well-balanced diet that meets their specific dietary demands by using cooking techniques that emphasize nutrient retention.

Short And Simple Recipes:

For those who have a colostomy, cooking healthy food quickly and easily is crucial to streamlining everyday activities and improving general health. Here are some delicious meals that are both nutrient-dense and easy to make:

1. Salad with Grilled Chicken:

- Ingredients: cucumber, cherry tomatoes, grilled chicken breast, mixed salad greens, and balsamic vinaigrette.

- Technique: Cook chicken breast on grill until done, then cut into strips. Combine with cucumber, cherry tomatoes, and fresh salad greens. Add a balsamic vinaigrette drizzle for a tasty yet light dinner.

2. Stir-fried vegetables:

- Ingredients: Sesame oil, low-sodium soy sauce, tofu or chicken strips, mixed veggies (bell peppers, broccoli, carrots, and snap peas).

- Technique: Sauté the desired protein and veggies in sesame oil until they are crisp-tender. For taste, add low-sodium soy sauce. Serve this quick and healthy stir-fry over brown rice.

3. Bowl of black beans with quinoa:

- Additions: Black beans, corn, avocado, cooked quinoa, cherry tomatoes, lime, and cilantro.

- Procedure: Put cooked quinoa, cherry tomatoes, diced avocado, black beans, and corn in a bowl. Add a squeeze of lime juice and some fresh cilantro as a garnish. This nutrient-dense bowl is simple to make and quite tasty.

4. Salmon baked with dill and lemon:

Salmon fillets, lemon slices, fresh dill, salt, and pepper are the ingredients.

- Technique: Arrange salmon fillets on a baking sheet, sprinkle with salt and pepper, and garnish with fresh dill and lemon slices. Bake the fish until it is well done. Patients with colostomies have a tasty and high-protein option in this easy meal.

These quick and simple dishes minimize the time and work needed in the kitchen while offering a range of flavors and nutrients. Including these dishes in a diet that is colostomy-friendly guarantees that people can eat appetizing and healthy food without endangering their digestive system.

CHAPTER ELEVEN

VITAMINS AND SUPPLEMENTS FOR PATIENTS WITH COLOSTOMY
Comprehending Nutritional Supplements

Supplemental nutrition is essential for maintaining the general health of those with colostomies. A piece of the colon is redirected to a hole in the abdominal wall during colostomy surgery, requiring dietary modifications. Promoting optimal health requires an understanding of the importance of dietary supplements in the context of colostomy treatment.

Patients with colostomies frequently experience difficulties absorbing nutrients because of changes to their digestive structures. As a result, the digestive tract may not absorb enough of several vital vitamins and minerals.

By giving concentrated quantities of these essential nutrients, nutritional supplements fill this gap and guarantee that the body gets what it needs to function properly.

Important vitamins and minerals for colostomy patients include calcium, iron, and zinc, as well as D, K, and S vitamins. Due to modifications in the digestive tract, B12, which is necessary for red blood cell production and neurological function, may be impaired in individuals with colostomies. Supplementing with vitamin D, which is essential for healthy bones, may be necessary, especially if exposure to sunshine is restricted. Sufficient consumption of calcium becomes essential to avoid problems with bone density, and iron supplements might be required to address any shortfalls that could result from changed nutrient absorption.

Furthermore, the anti-inflammatory properties of omega-3 fatty acids, which are present in fish oil supplements, may be advantageous for colostomy patients in treating inflammation-related issues. Probiotic pills may also help to minimize future problems like constipation by supporting digestion and preserving a healthy balance of gut flora.

Colostomy patients can make educated decisions about what they eat by being aware of the many functions of each nutritional supplement, which promotes maximum health and well-being.

The Value of Minerals and Vitamins

The human body requires vitamins and minerals to function properly, and the importance of these nutrients is increased for individuals who have colostomies. The anatomical changes brought about by colostomy surgery may affect how these vital nutrients are absorbed, so it is important to recognize their significance.

Vitamins are involved in many different physiological processes, each of which has a multitude of roles. For example, vitamin D plays a critical function in supporting bone health by being essential for the absorption of calcium. It can be difficult for colostomy patients to get enough vitamin D from sunshine exposure alone, so supplements are a useful way to avoid deficiencies.

Due to modifications in the digestive tract, vitamin B12, which is essential for red blood cell production and brain function, may be impaired in individuals with colostomies. This demonstrates how crucial taking B12 supplements is to preserving healthy health. Additionally, as vitamin K is essential for blood clotting, it must be taken into account to prevent consequences from impaired coagulation.

Minerals such as zinc, iron, and calcium are equally vital for colostomy patients. Calcium supplementation lowers the risk of bone density issues that may arise from changed nutrition absorption. When it comes to treating any deficits that can result in anemia, iron supplements become essential. Another necessary mineral, zinc, supports wound healing and immune system performance, two things that are very important for those recovering from surgery.

Understanding the significance of these vitamins and minerals enables colostomy patients to take charge of their dietary requirements proactively, promoting resilience and general health.

Speaking with Medical Experts

Engaging in professional consulting is essential for individualized and efficient care when pursuing a proactive colostomy diet. The structure of the digestive system is significantly altered after colostomy surgery, requiring a customized approach to meal planning.

Dietitians, nutritionists, and doctors are among the healthcare specialists who are essential in helping colostomy patients make the best nutritional decisions.

A medical expert can perform a thorough evaluation of the patient's nutritional state, accounting for variables including age, gender, previous medical histories, and the particulars of the colostomy procedure. This evaluation serves as the foundation for modifying dietary guidelines and locating any potential dietary gaps that might call for supplements.

Additionally, medical professionals can offer priceless advice on the selection and administration of particular dietary supplements. These experts' knowledge guarantees that colostomy patients are given reliable information, encouraging the prudent use of supplements without running the danger of overindulgence or negative side effects.

Frequent follow-up appointments enable the dietary plan to be modified in response to the patient's changing requirements and state of health. Healthcare providers can adjust recommendations and make sure the colostomy patient continues to receive enough nutrition for the best possible recovery and long-term health by tracking nutritional markers through blood tests and other evaluations.

In conclusion, creating a proactive colostomy diet that meets individual needs and promotes a healthy, balanced lifestyle requires cooperation between colostomy patients and medical specialists.

CHAPTER TWELVE

KEEPING YOUR BOWEL MOVEMENTS REGULAR
Dietary Fiber and the Placenta:

Maintaining regular bowel motions is mostly dependent on diet, particularly for those who have a colostomy. One important factor that has a big impact on digestive health and can help with smoother bowel movements is dietary fiber. The indigestible part of plant meals called fiber gives feces more volume, facilitates passage through the digestive system, and encourages regular bowel movements. It's critical to comprehend how dietary fiber affects the digestive system of people who have colostomies.

Constipation and diarrhea can be avoided by including a sufficient amount of dietary fiber in the colostomy diet. Selecting soluble fiber sources is crucial because they can absorb water and solidify into a gel-like substance that softens and facilitates the passage of stool. Examples of such sources include legumes, oats, and some fruits. Whole grains, vegetables, and nuts include insoluble fiber, which gives feces more volume and facilitates a quicker passage through the digestive system.

After colostomy surgery, it is important to gradually add fiber to the diet. Bloating, gas, or discomfort may result from abrupt increases in fiber consumption. When taking fiber, it's equally crucial to stay hydrated as this promotes optimal function and guards against potential problems.

Moreover, certain fiber-rich food types that may result in gas or odor should be avoided by those who have a colostomy. Making a customized and well-tolerated diet plan can benefit from keeping a food journal and recording how various fiber sources influence bowel motions.

Through knowledge of the subtleties of dietary fiber and adjusting consumption to suit specific requirements, people who have colostomies can improve their overall quality of life by promoting a more comfortable and predictable bowel habit.

Foods that Encourage Regular Urinary Movements:

Making the correct meal choices is crucial for colostomy patients who want to continue having regular bowel movements. Certain foods contain qualities that can facilitate digestion, stave against constipation, and improve intestinal health in general. A well-balanced and successful colostomy diet can be achieved by including a range of nutrient-rich foods in the diet.

The main components of a diet that encourages regular bowel motions are fruits and vegetables. They supply vital vitamins, minerals, and fiber—all of which are important for maintaining intestinal health. Because of their high soluble fiber content, berries, apples, and pears in particular help to soften stool and stave against constipation. Broccoli, carrots, and leafy greens are good sources of insoluble fiber that help move stool through the digestive system and increase its volume.

Whole grains are great sources of fiber and can help maintain regular bowel movements. Whole wheat, quinoa, and brown rice are a few types of whole grains. By giving feces more volume, these grains improve digestive health and offer long-lasting energy.

It's important to be aware of any trigger foods that could upset your stomach or affect how your stools smell. Some people may need to limit their intake of particular spices, dairy products, or high-fiber foods, or avoid them completely.

A diet that supports regular bowel movements and healthy digestive function can be created by individuals with colostomies by choosing a varied variety of nutrient-dense foods and considering individual tolerances.

Keeping An Eye On And Modifying Fiber Intake:

For people with colostomies, achieving and sustaining regularity in bowel movements necessitates a proactive approach to monitoring and modifying fiber intake. While a healthy diet is necessary for digestive health, constipation, and diarrhea can be avoided by striking the correct balance.

A useful tactic is to maintain an extensive food journal where you record the kinds and quantities of foods high in fiber that you eat, as well as how they affect your bowel movements. Informed modifications may be made thanks to the identification of patterns and connections between nutrition and digestive function through this method. It is best to gradually introduce new foods and monitor the digestive system's reaction, particularly following colostomy surgery.

Keeping an eye on hydration is another aspect of tracking fiber consumption. Drinking enough water is essential for the digestive system's fiber to work properly. Fiber softens stools and facilitates their easy passage by absorbing water. It is important to emphasize the connection between fiber and fluid consumption because dehydration can result in issues like constipation.

Seeking advice from a medical practitioner or a certified nutritionist is crucial if constipation or diarrhea doesn't go away after dietary changes. They may guarantee that the person's nutritional requirements are satisfied, offer tailored advice, and suggest certain dietary adjustments.

Colostomy patients can actively control their digestive health, encouraging regular bowel movements and improving their general well-being, by taking an alert and flexible attitude to their fiber intake.

CHAPTER THIRTEEN

ADVICE FOR COLOSTOMY PATIENTS TRAVELING
Making Travel Plans in Advance:

When starting a journey, colostomy sufferers must plan everything out carefully. When traveling with a colostomy, it's important to plan for any obstacles and put strategies in place to make sure everything goes smoothly. Learning about the amenities and medical facilities at the location is one of the first stages in preparation. Doing some research on local pharmacies and hospitals gives you peace of mind and guarantees that you'll have access to the resources you need in an emergency.

It is also imperative that restroom breaks and rest stops be factored into the itinerary. Finding accessible private or public restrooms can reduce worry and guarantee comfort while traveling. Patients who have a colostomy may find it helpful to schedule their trip around times of the day when their digestive systems are normally less active, which will lessen the need for frequent bathroom breaks.

Additionally, making ahead arrangements with hotels, airlines, or other transportation providers might help to ensure a more comfortable trip. Notifying them of particular requirements, such as the need for extra medical supplies or the need to take ostomy equipment through security checks, guarantees that the required preparations are made.

Packing Necessities:

Colostomy patients need to pack carefully for travel, putting up a complete kit that meets their unique requirements. An adequate supply of skin barriers, disposal bags, adhesive removers, and ostomy pouches are essential items. In case of unanticipated delays or emergencies, it is recommended to have extra supplies that can last for several days.

Keeping a small, travel-sized ostomy kit with scissors, wipes, and a changing mat with you makes changing your pouches unobtrusive and hygienic. It's crucial to carry enough comfortable apparel in addition to medical necessities. When traveling for extended periods, loose-fitting clothing composed of breathable fabric can assist reduce irritation and increase comfort.

Another essential item for colostomy patients is a travel-friendly water bottle, which helps them stay hydrated during their trip. Sustaining an appropriate fluid intake is essential because dehydration can worsen problems associated with ostomy management. It's also convenient to have prescription drugs and any necessary medical records in carry-on luggage for quick access in case of emergency medical crises or security inspections.

Managing Techniques When Traveling:

Adapting coping mechanisms is necessary when traveling with a colostomy to handle the emotional and physical demands of the trip. Keeping an optimistic outlook and viewing the trip as an opportunity for adventure rather than a cause of worry is one useful tactic. Travel-related anxiety can be reduced by practicing relaxation techniques like deep breathing or meditation.

Colostomy patients also need to be aware of their body's signals and take breaks when necessary. Including these breaks in the travel schedule, whether it be for a quick stroll, some quiet time for contemplation, or just finding a cozy place to relax, can greatly improve general well-being.

Furthermore, using common sense and prudence can be helpful coping strategies. Being flexible is essential when traveling because unforeseen circumstances can occur. To ensure a helpful and understanding atmosphere, colostomy patients should feel empowered to openly convey their needs to travel companions, airline staff, and lodging providers.

To sum up, early preparation, cautious packing, and useful coping mechanisms are the cornerstones of a good trip for colostomy patients. People with colostomies can confidently travel the world and prioritize their health and well-being by including these components in their travel routines.

CHAPTER FOURTEEN

TYPICAL PROBLEMS AND THEIR FIXES
Handling Digestive Problems

A common aspect of proactive colostomy eating is overcoming the different digestive obstacles that can come from altered anatomy and alterations in stool function after colostomy surgery. Gas, bloating, constipation, or diarrhea are among the problems that people with colostomies may experience. These problems can negatively affect the quality of their life. A multifaceted approach involving dietary alterations, hydration techniques, and lifestyle improvements is necessary to manage these intestinal issues.

One of the main things to do is keep an eye on the foods you choose to find triggers that make digestive issues worse. Some foods, such as those high in fiber, might exacerbate bloating or cause gas production to increase. As a result, people may need to carefully introduce new foods into their diets while keeping an eye on how their bodies react. Furthermore, chewing food well helps facilitate digestion and lessen the chance of pain.

Hydration is essential for colostomy patients to preserve the health of their digestive systems. Consuming enough water aids in preventing constipation, which is a prevalent issue in this demographic. Finding the ideal mix is crucial, though, as consuming too much fluids might aggravate diarrhea. It's crucial to keep an eye on each person's hydration requirements and modify intake as necessary.

In addition to dietary changes, engaging in regular exercise helps support a healthy digestive system. Exercise helps avoid constipation and encourages bowel movements.

To receive individualized advice, people should speak with healthcare providers and adjust their exercise regimen to their unique health situation.

In addition, psychological issues that could be linked to digestive issues must be addressed. Anxiety and stress can affect the digestive tract and exacerbate symptoms. Deep breathing exercises, mindfulness, and soothing activities are some of the techniques that can help manage stress and support improved digestive health.

To sum up, proactive colostomy dieting for digestive problems requires a multifaceted strategy that includes food adjustments, proper hydration, frequent exercise, and psychological counseling. It is advised that people collaborate closely with medical specialists to customize plans to meet their specific requirements and enhance their general health.

Resolving Nutritional Issues

Those who decide to start a proactive colostomy diet may need to address several dietary issues that may come up as they become used to a new eating routine. These worries include controlling weight, making sure you're getting enough nutrition, and dealing with the particular food restrictions that the colostomy itself places on you. To overcome these obstacles, nutritional planning, and execution must be done with consideration and individuality.

Making sure you are getting enough nutrition even with dietary restrictions is one of the main things to think about. Nutrient absorption may be impacted by colostomy surgery, thus patients may need to closely monitor their diet to avoid deficits. It becomes essential to seek advice from a registered dietitian or other healthcare provider to create a meal plan that is both individualized and nutritionally balanced. This strategy may include changes or supplements to guarantee sufficient consumption of vital vitamins and minerals.

Further areas of attention in diagnosing and treating dietary issues are calorie consumption and weight control. After colostomy surgery, some people may have weight swings. It is important to maintain a healthy weight for general well-being. It becomes essential to balance the amount of calories consumed with physical activity, and depending on lifestyle circumstances and individual metabolic rates, modifications may be required.

Another layer of complexity is the dietary limitations associated with the colostomy itself, such as avoiding specific foods that may irritate or cause clogs. To do this, a detailed study of the person's digestive system is necessary, as is some experimentation with different foods to find possible triggers. Making a list of foods that are acceptable and unbearable will help you make better nutritional decisions.

Troubleshooting nutritional issues also heavily depends on meal planning and preparation. Meal planning may be helpful for people, with an emphasis on smaller, more frequent meals and readily digested foods. While taking into account dietary restrictions and individual tastes, incorporating a range of textures and flavors can improve the entire dining experience.

To sum up, diagnosing nutritional issues in proactive colostomy dieting is a thorough process that takes into account meal planning, weight control, dietary restrictions, and nutritional requirements. Working together with medical experts guarantees that people receive tailored advice, promoting an effective and long-lasting approach to their dietary journey.

Seeking Expert Advice

Setting out on a proactive path of colostomy diets requires working in tandem with medical specialists who can offer invaluable advice, support, and knowledge. Seeking expert advice is essential for colostomy patients to navigate the challenges of managing digestive issues, making dietary adjustments, and maintaining their general well-being.

An expert in gastrointestinal health and a licensed dietician is one of the most important professional resources on this trip. These professionals have the expertise to customize dietary advice to meet the needs of each individual, taking into account things like the kind of colostomy, dietary limitations, and any underlying medical issues. A dietitian can help people manage their weight, maximize their nutrient intake, and take care of digestive issues with evidence-based dietary practices.

Gastroenterologists and colorectal surgeons are also essential in offering expert advice. Frequent follow-up appointments enable the surgery site to be monitored, bowel function to be assessed, and any new issues or concerns to be discussed. People can receive timely advice, care plan revisions, and appropriate interventions to address difficulties swiftly when they have open communication with these healthcare experts.

Holistic coaching is enhanced by the involvement of mental health professionals and support groups in addition to medical professionals. People can get emotional support from peers who understand the particular difficulties of living with a colostomy by joining a support group and sharing stories and helpful advice. Psychologists and counselors are examples of mental health specialists who can assist people in managing the emotional aspects of transitioning to life with a colostomy by addressing issues like anxiety, body image, and self-esteem.

In conclusion, collaborating with a multidisciplinary team that includes registered dietitians, colorectal surgeons, gastroenterologists, and mental health specialists is necessary when seeking professional advice on proactive colostomy dieting. This method guarantees all-encompassing care, attends to specific requirements, and equips people to face the obstacles of having a colostomy with self-assurance and fortitude.

CHAPTER FIFTEEN

HONORING WELL-BEING AND HEALTH
Considering the Advancement:

An essential part of celebrating your health and fitness is taking stock of your colostomy diet journey. Through self-reflection, people can evaluate their accomplishments, recognize obstacles they have conquered, and notice gains in their general well-being. Reflecting for a moment increases one's sense of accomplishment and gives you the drive to continue following a proactive colostomy eating plan.

When it comes to colostomy dieting, reflection frequently entails going over food selections, keeping an eye on digestive processes, and recording any changes in energy levels. This is a chance to commemorate effective dietary changes that have improved digestive health and, in turn, general quality of life. Realizing that they may adjust and modify their diet to ensure improved nutritional absorption and digestive comfort may make people happy.

Furthermore, considering advancements extends beyond the physical facets of well-being. It also includes the psychological and emotional aspects. Colostomy surgery can have a significant effect on mental health, thus it's important to evaluate coping mechanisms and emotional resilience. Holistic health greatly benefits from appreciating the capacity to overcome emotional obstacles and keep an optimistic outlook.

Essentially, the process of reviewing one's progress allows people to maintain a sense of connection with their health journey, thereby highlighting the significance of their efforts. It provides the groundwork for ongoing development, fostering resiliency and a forward-thinking outlook for the future.

Goal-setting for Long-Term Health:

Proactive colostomy nutrition guidelines must include the essential component of setting long-term health goals. It gives people a road map for long-term well-being, giving their food choices and way of life focus and direction. A comprehensive approach to treating a colostomy is ensured by setting specific and achievable long-term health goals, which promote overall physical and mental wellness.

When it comes to colostomy dieting, long-term health objectives frequently entail developing eating patterns that promote ideal digestive function, reduce the risk of problems, and improve absorption of nutrients. A wide variety of nutrient-dense diets, controlling hydration levels, and gradually introducing new foods to gauge their effect on digestive comfort are a few examples of these objectives.

Furthermore, long-term health objectives go beyond dietary guidelines. They include lifestyle decisions like consistent exercise, stress reduction, and enough sleep that support general wellness. By addressing the interrelated facets of well-being, the incorporation of these components into a holistic health plan promotes a proactive approach to colostomy treatment.

Establishing attainable deadlines and benchmarks is essential for creating long-term health objectives. With this method, people can monitor their development, acknowledge their accomplishments along the way, and modify their colostomy diet plan as needed. In the end, setting and achieving long-term health objectives offers a framework for a happy and healthy existence as well as a sense of purpose and motivation.

<u>**Accepting a Lifestyle of Proactivity:**</u>

The cornerstone of long-term health and fitness for people managing a colostomy is adopting a proactive lifestyle. Taking deliberate, preventative action to maximize one's physical, emotional, and mental well-being is known as a proactive approach. It emphasizes on creating routines and habits that lead to a happy and fulfilled life rather than only responding to health issues.

Adopting a proactive lifestyle in the context of colostomy dieting entails continuously making educated food decisions, being aware of the body's signals, and being proactive in handling any obstacles that may arise. This entails being in constant contact with medical staff, remaining up to date on developments in colostomy care, and actively engaging in one's healthcare process.

Developing an optimistic outlook is essential to living a proactive lifestyle. Colostomy patients may have particular difficulties; adopting a proactive mentality entails seeing these difficulties as chances for development and adaptation. This resilience improves the capacity to manage the emotional implications of having a colostomy and contributes to general mental health.

A proactive lifestyle also includes self-care routines that support mental and physical equilibrium. This can entail doing frequent, capacity-appropriate exercise, practicing mindfulness to reduce stress, and taking part in joyful and fulfilling pursuits. People can celebrate the resiliency of the human spirit and lay the groundwork for long-term health by incorporating these practices into their daily lives.

Adopting a proactive lifestyle within the framework of colostomy diets is essentially a dedication to holistic well-being and personal empowerment. Despite the difficulties a colostomy presents, it is a deliberate decision to actively participate in one's health journey to promote a feeling of control, purpose, and celebration of life.